To

Thank you for being there for me. your guidance has been very helpfull, and I am forever grateful, Thankyou

with love,

FINDING THE LIGHT WITHIN

Finding The Light Within

Tanner Bergsma

Contents

Dedication   vii
REMEMBER   ix

1	Where It All Began	1
2	The Stars are Brighter in the darkness	7
3	When Trust Becomes a Weapon	13
4	Running on Empty	15
5	The Chains of Bondage	23
6	Finding A Glimmer of Hope	33
7	Building Something Bigger	43
8	The Lessons I Learned	51
9	Pain into Purpose	61
10	Lack of Self Love	69
11	Legacy	81

About the Author   90

Copyright © 2024 by Tanner Bergsma
All rights reserved. No part of this book may be reproduced in any manner whatsoever without written permission except in the case of brief quotations embodied in critical articles and reviews.
First Printing, 2024

This book is dedicated to all those who have stood by me, believed in me, and lifted me up when I needed it most.
To the people and humanity at large—may this book serve as a reminder of our shared strength, resilience, and limitless potential. And to anyone who has ever faced adversity, know this: you are capable of achieving anything you set your mind to. This book is for you.
With deepest gratitude and hope,

Tanner Bergsma

REMEMBER

"Strength isn't found in avoiding the fall - it's in rising every time we do. Keep going, because every setback builds the bridge to the life you're meant to live."

Tanner Bergsma

1

Where It All Began

It's hard to find the right words to capture the weight of my past. Writing this brings back the flood of tears and pain I've carried, and as I look back at my life, I'm overwhelmed by the memories. Many people face homelessness for countless reasons, but my story is different. It wasn't what you might expect. As I write, I can only share my perspective—the way I felt in those moments and the scars I still bear today.

I grew up in the small city of Stratford, Ontario. My childhood is mostly a blur. I've come to realize it's because I had to block out so much of what happened. Talking about it is difficult because some people may try to defend themselves instead of facing the truth. But the truth is, in my early years, I experienced a level of abuse and neglect that no child should endure. I'm not here to point fingers—I've worked hard to find healing and let go of blame. Still, the reality is that I almost didn't make it through. The pain I faced nearly killed me. High school was a nightmare. I was bullied relentlessly, mocked for being different, and pushed into deeper isolation. I wasn't the kind of person who could shrug it off. The weight of it all crushed me, and I tried to disappear—sitting alone at lunch or avoiding people altogether. Inside, I was screaming for help, crying myself to sleep most nights.

When I was thirteen, Family and Children's Services got involved. They were supposed to help, but instead, they made things worse. Their words, their actions—they didn't heal me. They cut me deeper. I still carry the wounds of their empty promises and manipulations. My pain was twisted into their narrative, and I was left unheard, invisible, drowning.

I tried to speak up, but no one listened. Not when I cried out, not when I self-harmed, not even when I was suicidal. Everyone seemed too busy defending themselves to see what was happening to me. The home I lived in became suffocating—a place of endless arguments and chaos. I felt trapped, like I was reliving the same hellish day over and over. The fear was so intense that I slept with a knife under my pillow, locking my door every night just to feel a sliver of safety. The pain was relentless. I was trapped within a mental prison. It wasn't just emotional—it was physical, like being stabbed again and again with a scorching shive. My soul felt shredded, and I didn't know how to stop the bleeding. Eventually, I couldn't take it anymore. I ran away—not just to escape the pain, but to protect the fragile ties I had with my family. Even now, I can't bring myself to share everything. The memories are too raw, the trauma too deep.

Complex PTSD clouds my past, and I can only revisit pieces of it at a time. Looking back, I'm amazed I survived. I yearned for love, only to be pushed aside, beaten down, and trampled on. Yet here I am, piecing together my story one shard at a time, trying to make sense of the brokenness I've carried for so long.

The day came when I couldn't take it anymore. I ran away, slipping through the back hedge with nothing but socks on my feet, a t-shirt, and a pair of jeans. It was late June, around 6 p.m., and the evening air carried the weight of my desperation. Countless times before, I had tried to escape, only to be dragged back into the mental prison that was my life. This time, I was determined. For a few days, I hid in the shadows of Stratford's corridors, unsure of what to do next. My heart ached, my spirit screamed for freedom, and yet, deep inside, a spark flared—something raw, something stubborn. It drove me forward. On the third day, I decided to walk to Waterloo, a city I had only imagined, hoping it held the promise of a fresh start.

I began my journey on the side of Highway 8 West, leaving from Ontario Street. The pavement stretched endlessly ahead of me, and each step sent pain searing through my feet, raw and swollen from hours of walking in flimsy flip-flops. The ache was unbearable, like walking on burning coals. Still, I pressed on.

Every step was a battle, but my dream of university pushed me through the torment. I couldn't stop—I wouldn't stop. After what felt like an eternity, I reached New Hamburg, my legs trembling with exhaustion. Outside a Mc-

Donald's by the No Frills, I found myself at the drive-thru, desperate for water. That's when a stranger pulled up and offered to buy me food. I was too weak to say no. We sat on a bench, and as he handed me the food, my walls crumbled. The tears I had fought so hard to hide spilled over. I told him my story—why I had run, why I was walking this impossible road. He listened, truly listened. Before we parted, he suggested I speak to factory workers heading home to Waterloo.

With new resolve, I approached cars leaving the factory. Most people turned me away, but eventually, an older man in his fifties offered me a ride. He didn't ask for much, just dropped me off by Laurier University. By then, it was 4:30 a.m. The cold bit into my skin, and I was utterly alone.

The streets offered no comfort. Rain drizzled down as the bitter June night wrapped me in its icy grip. I wandered aimlessly until I found a patch of trees near the train tracks in Uptown Waterloo. Curling up under their sparse cover, I tried to shield myself from the elements, but sleep wouldn't come. It was a brutal, sleepless night, and there would be many more like it. For two long weeks, this was my life—cold, wet, and hungry. My body grew weaker, but I forced myself to keep moving. Then, one day, I met Antonio. He was a tall, thin man in his thirties, a Colombian with an easy smile and a sharp mind. Though he was struggling too, Antonio knew the city's resources inside and out.

We spent time together, and his kindness gave me a sliver of hope. He told me about a men's shelter in Kitchener. When I arrived, they referred me to One Roof Youth

Services. I walked through those doors with nothing but the clothes on my back and a head full of questions.

2

The Stars are Brighter in the darkness

After my initial intake at the youth shelter, I found myself amongst the other homeless youth. It was my first time being on my own with other people my age. It was strange at first. But the youth there were not afraid to express themselves. One youth, her name was Stewart, she was a trans female who was very outspoken and confident. We quickly became close friends. She was tall for her age, thin, and always liked to present herself in the best clothes she could. She was dating a guy at the time; his name was Alex. Alex and I became close friends almost instantly. Alex is not the type of person you would expect to be homeless. You can tell he had good parents, but he was adopted. He would often do outlandishly stupid things just for the fun of it, and liked to make them into adventures. He called it "Stoney ventures." So, we used to go on these so called 'stoney ventures' which often would be the group of us, Stu,

Alex, Zack (a close friend of Alex's), and me. We would often go down to Rockway in Kitchener or to the park. One venture he took us on was to Uptown Waterloo at night, and whoever found the cheapest weed in the city won. It was a funny sight. Another time he would hang around with a guy named Nick, (who often got in trouble for stealing cars), and we'd all go in this car with him and Nick would sit shotgun and would have fun smoking while driving to the reserve to get more. I never knew that the car was of course stolen, and was too naive about remembering the dangers about anything. Later turned out that they were making drug runs the whole time, with me in the car. Now I was luckily not around when they got busted, but I was hanging out with the wrong crowd a lot just to fit in as that was the 'cool thing' to do. Never started smoking before then, but ever since hanging out with them I constantly would smoke and drink and do weed. But at the end of almost every day, when everyone else was asleep, Alex and I would head outside late at night to go on walks with Zack. Usually was to the Short Stop convenience store just to get smokes for Alex and lottery tickets for Zack. We then would often go to Rockway where we would sometimes just sit and relax with the other youth (which I called Roofies and the name stuck). Often, we would lay on the grass and look up at the stars, most roofies wasted out of their minds. I never was intoxicated, and just wanted to fit in. I laid down and I too often looked at the stars, reflecting back on my life. I would often wonder how I was going to get back on my feet. Or I was reflecting back on my life. Or even sometimes my dreams in life. Somehow the stars made my problems all go away. The twinkling of the stars made me warm up from the inside. It was the only thing keeping me from ending my life. All I knew is that if I was going to survive, I had to do something and quick.

Finding my first place to live felt like a challenging puzzle to solve. I completed applications and attended viewings, but many landlords rejected me as soon as they heard the phrase "youth shelter." I recall entering a rooming house one day, holding tightly to the small amount of cash I had saved, wondering, perhaps this is the moment. The landlord, a rough-around-the-edges guy with the lingering scent of cigarette smoke, looked at me with a hint of skepticism but eventually gave me the keys after a brief talk about the importance of timely rent payments. It may have been small—a little room with worn walls and one window—but it was my own. I sensed a glimmer of hope that perhaps I was beginning to move towards something better.

During that period, I was able to secure a position with a duct cleaning company. It may not have been glamorous, but that paycheck was essential for making ends meet. Nemar, my boss, was swift in bringing me on board, emphasizing that his company truly appreciates dedicated individuals. Initially, I found myself admiring him. He appeared warm and engaging, possessing a manner of speaking that put others at comfort. He welcomed me into his circle, frequently giving me the simpler tasks and guiding me through the process.

But as the days went by, his "kindness" began to seem less sincere. He started making remarks that seemed a bit strange—compliments that hung in the air a bit too long, inquiries about my personal life that felt too probing. I attempted to let it go. I really needed this job. But one evening, everything shifted.

It was a late shift, just the two of us wrapping up a job in a client's home. We finished cleaning the air ducts and were packing up the equipment when he casually asked if I wanted to grab a drink. I kindly said no, explaining that I was feeling tired and wanted to head home. That's when he cornered me, his smile fading, replaced by an unsettling intensity.

He began with words that seemed like compliments, yet there was an underlying sharpness that unsettled me. As I attempted to pull away, he took hold of my arm. "Don't hold back," he said, his voice calm and steady. I stood still, thoughts swirling in my head. I had been unaware of many things in the past, but at that moment, everything became clear to me.

I found a way to step back, quietly saying I needed to use the bathroom. As soon as he couldn't see me anymore, I took out my phone and acted like I was on a call, speaking loudly about someone coming to get me. When I returned to the room, his demeanor had reverted to its insincere kindness, yet I could sense his gaze on me as I gathered the remaining gear.

The following days at work felt incredibly difficult. He began to make veiled threats, cautioning me not to "misunderstand" what he meant. He suggested that he had control over my job security and my ability to pay my rent. The impact of those words felt overwhelming.

In the end, I reached my limit. I stepped away from the job, fully aware that I would be giving up the small income I had. I just couldn't remain in that atmosphere. I realized I had swapped one form of struggle for another, finding myself in the same place—alone, without money, and uncertain about my next steps.

Reflecting on that experience, I learned so much about what it means to endure. It wasn't merely about securing food or shelter—it was about understanding the dangers that exploit weakness. It was about discovering the courage to step away, even when the other option felt equally disheartening.

Healing from what happened with Nemar was a long journey for me. There are still times when the memory slips in, unexpected. I keep reminding myself that I made it through. I decided to stand up for myself, even when it seemed like everything was working against me.

Perhaps, in a unique way, those stars I once gazed upon were indeed correct. There was a strength within me that I hadn't fully acknowledged. A force that kept me going, even when the night felt its darkest.

3

When Trust Becomes a Weapon

Life often intertwines the essence of survival with the openness of vulnerability. I believed I had discovered a sense of stability in a place I could call home, yet having a roof above me didn't guarantee my safety. The room I rented was supposed to be a peaceful retreat, but it turned into a struggle—one where I felt defeated. I allowed my former friend to stay at my place because I understood the feeling of having nowhere to turn. He appeared to be in a tough spot, and I felt a sense of trust towards him. He had his flaws, that's true, but I was completely unaware of what I was bringing into my life. He never mentioned that he was using meth and fentanyl, but it became clear pretty quickly. His behavior changed unpredictably—one moment he was calm, and the next he was filled with a frantic energy that made my stomach churn with unease.

It occurred one night after I explained to him that he needed to leave. He reacted poorly to it. His laughter felt empty, and his eyes, frantic and red, pierced through me. He called me a traitor, his voice growing louder, his presence feeling more imposing with every moment that went by. Before I even had a chance to respond, he had me pinned down and pulled down my pants.

I made an effort to resist, but he overpowered me, his force amplified by the substances flowing in his system. My voice faltered—screams trapped within me as I grappled with the terrifying truth of what was unfolding. I felt a deep sense of vulnerability, my body not responding as he took control, his grip unyielding.

Once it ended, I felt disconnected from myself. The walls of my room, which used to offer a bit of solace, now seemed to tighten around me, becoming more oppressive with each moment that passed. I scrubbed my body in the shower, but no amount of soap could wash away the heaviness I felt inside.

Just when I thought I could finally catch my breath and consider moving on, it happened once more.

4

Running on Empty

After she left, I returned to the streets, where all that truly mattered was survival. The isolation felt overwhelming. I found myself alone, exposed to the chill without any shelter. All that I had worked tirelessly to create was lost, taking with it the delicate sense of stability I had held onto.

Life on the streets is real and unyielding. It takes away your sense of dignity and makes you exist from one moment to the next, constantly on edge, anticipating the next hit. One night, as I was walking in search of shelter, I felt a sudden impact.

I took a turn into an alley, hoping it would lead me to a quicker path. A man stepped out from the darkness; his gun pointed directly at my chest. His voice carried a calm and unwavering quality. "Show me what you've got," he said. I stood still, feeling my heart race in my chest. I really didn't have much—just a handful of crumpled bills and my phone. But he was indifferent. He took it all, leaving me with just the clothes I was wearing.

That moment transformed something within me. It wasn't only the fear; it was the feeling of being powerless. The streets had transformed into more than just a means of getting by; they had become a battleground, and I found myself ill-equipped for the fight.

Before long, I was gathered with a few others who were also without homes, finding comfort in each other's presence. One of them was my best friend, a person I've shared countless memories with over the years. We had shared countless experiences, and my trust in him was deeper than with anyone else. He had been facing challenges with addiction for quite a while, and life on the streets had only intensified those struggles.

One night, he took too much right in front of me. I will always remember how his body went limp, how his lips turned blue. I felt a rush of anxiety as I fumbled with the Narcan I had with me for emergencies. I felt a tremor in my hands as I gave it, hoping with all my heart that it would be effective. After what seemed like forever, he took a deep breath and returned to the world. A wave of relief came over me, but it didn't last long.

His struggle with addiction created ongoing tension, ultimately resulting in a clash with a local gang. He had a significant debt to them, and when he was unable to settle it, they shifted their focus onto me. They viewed me as someone vulnerable, a person they could manipulate to convey their point.

One night, they surrounded us, revealing their true intentions. "You're both finished," one of them said with a mocking tone, holding a knife menacingly. My friend and I had a close call. That was the moment I realized I had to make a change. I just had to leave.

I escaped to Listowel, a quaint little town where I thought I could blend in and begin anew. But Listowel didn't turn out to be the safe haven I had envisioned. I found myself homeless, struggling to get by, but now I was in a new and unfamiliar environment. The nights felt chillier, the streets more subdued, yet the burden of all I had faced lingered with me.

I frequently took a moment to think about the distance I had come from where I once was. From being married and dreaming of a secure future to losing everything and fleeing for my life—it felt like I was stuck in a nightmare with no escape. The betrayal, the robbery, the overdose, the threats—each of these experiences had etched deep scars that refused to fade.

Yet, even in the toughest times, a glimmer of hope remained. I reminded myself that as long as I continued to move forward and take each breath, there remained a possibility for something greater. It may not have been a lot, but it was sufficient to motivate me.

Listowel became a significant part of my journey, challenging my strength and resilience in ways I never expected. This wasn't the conclusion of my journey; it was simply another chapter, a reminder that no matter how deep the fall, there's always a path to rise once more.

In Listowel, I soon discovered that small towns can be lively places, full of unexpected energy. Experiencing homelessness in such an environment can feel incredibly lonely. There were no busy city shelters or outreach programs, no lively sidewalks where you could blend in with the crowd. You're simply present, visible to all, without any protection.

I began staying with friends, moving from one home to the next. Every stop seemed fleeting, and indeed it was. Some couches were offered with a sense of pity, while others came with a reluctant air, as if there was an unspoken hope that my stay would be brief. It was tough for me to reach out for help, but I felt like I had no other option.

Days seamlessly flowed into weeks. I realized I was feeling exhausted, not only in my body but also in my spirit. Homelessness carries a weight that influences every choice, all centered on the need to survive. Where will I be resting tonight? What should I eat tomorrow? Will I truly discover a path beyond this?

Then, on a regular day, my phone buzzed with a message that completely changed everything for me. A friend casually shared that my daughter had come into the world. I stood still.

"Which daughter are you referring to?" I replied, feeling a slight tremor in my hands.

I wasn't informed, and I had no idea she had even come into the world. I reflected on the months that had passed, remembering the fractured bond with her mother. Although we hadn't separated on the best note, I still held onto the hope of being a part of my child's life. That hope now feels broken, leaving a deep emptiness in my chest.

I felt a sense of helplessness. Who was she, really? How was she as a person? Is she alright? Thoughts swirled in my head, yet clarity eluded me. The news hit hard, almost like a harsh reality check.

Weeks passed, and her presence lingered in my mind. Regardless of the circumstances, I felt a strong desire to support her. I felt a strong desire to connect with her, to embrace the role of a father, even though I was unsure of the way forward. But what could I give her when I felt empty inside?

Then the call arrived that would transform everything.

I found myself in a coffee shop, connecting to the Wi-Fi to search for job opportunities and figuring out my next steps. My phone rang. I received a call from my ex. Usually, I would have let it go, but for some reason, I felt compelled to answer.

"Hey there?" I spoke with care.

"Is this Tanner?" my ex's voice inquired.

"Yes," I said, feeling a mix of curiosity and openness.

"Hey Tanner it's me. I just thought I'd let you know that I gave birth four days ago. I am in the hospital now at Grand River. Myla has been rushed off to McMaster Hospital due to her fragile state."

My heart skipped a beat. For a moment, I felt completely overwhelmed.

"What is going on?" I was able to get the words out.

"She is not doing well... but you can go visit her if you want."

I chose not to seek an explanation. I got a lift from a friend and hurried to the hospital as quickly as possible. I felt a whirlwind of ideas swirling in my head. Did she get hurt in labor? Was she unwell? What the hell was going on?

Upon my arrival, a nurse led me to a room where my small, delicate baby rested in her incubator. She looked extremely beautiful. More beautiful than I could have ever imagined. She was small though. Like Extremely small. The nurse shared that there were some complications following her birth, and that her mother had entrusted her to the hospital's care.

I experienced a whirlwind of emotions that were hard to grasp—joy, fear, love, guilt. This little one, so beautifully delicate and pure, belonged to me. Even with all that I had faced and my imperfections, she was present, and she relied on me. I wasn't sure how it would happen, but I made a promise to myself and to her that I would figure it out. I was determined to be the father she truly deserved, no matter what it took.

In that moment, as I stood in the sterile hospital room and gazed at my daughter for the first time, everything changed in a way I never anticipated. Life has thrown its challenges my way, yet she has inspired me to keep pushing forward.

After a long while, I found myself feeling hopeful. It's not about me; it's about her. She represented my opportunity to reshape my narrative, to improve myself, to overcome all that had sought to bring me down.

5

The Chains of Bondage

The call arrived in the stillness of the night, shattering the fragile peace that lingered in the air. I found myself curled up on a stranger's couch, utterly drained from yet another day spent desperately trying to mend the shattered fragments of my life in Listowel. The sudden buzz of my phone shattered the stillness, a jarring reminder of everything I've lost. I paused, an overwhelming weight pressing down on my heart.

"This is McMaster Hospital," the voice said when I picked up, sending a chill through my heart. "Your daughter is gravely unwell." "You have to come right now."

My heart sank. I felt suffocated, my mind a fog of despair. "What do you mean, sick?" What is happening? I pleaded, my voice quaking with despair.

"She's in a critical state," the voice whispered, heavy with despair. "Please, you have to come right away."

I hung up, my heart aching, and immediately dialed my ex. My hands trembled uncontrollably, and I found myself struggling to press the right buttons, needing three attempts to get it right. When she picked up, I couldn't hold back the words that spilled from my heart, raw and unfiltered, revealing the pain I had just discovered. She said she would rush to the hospital immediately.

"I'll meet you there," I said, my heart heavy with uncertainty, though I had no idea how I'd find my way to that place without you.

The next hour felt like a whirlwind of despair. I cried out desperately, hoping that someone, anyone, would hear my pleas and help me reach Hamilton. It felt as though the world around me was shrouded in a heavy silence, with most people either lost in their dreams or completely unaware of the pain that lingered in the air. It was as if my cries were swallowed by an endless emptiness. With each passing moment, my heart ached deeper as I envisioned my precious daughter, isolated and fighting her battles all alone. At last, someone reluctantly offered to drive me, but it came after a painful struggle. The ride is a haze, a fleeting memory overshadowed by the suffocating heaviness that clings to my heart. Each passing minute dragged on, stretching into an endless ache.

When I finally got there, it was already 1:30 in the morning. Seeing her there shattered me, and the expression on her face revealed all the painful truths I wished to avoid. My daughter, my precious and delicate daughter, was slipping away from me. She was just a fragile eight days old.

The nurse guided me into the NICU, a cold, sterile room drenched in harsh white light, where the relentless beeping of machines and the soft, sorrowful hum of ventilators filled the air. My heart shattered as I gazed upon her fragile form, ensnared by a web of wires and tubes. She appeared so fragile, so lost, as if she were out of place in this harsh and unfeeling environment.

But then I caught a glimpse of them. The nurses. They stood by her incubator, their laughter echoing in the hollow space, a stark contrast to the heaviness in my heart. Crying.

My heart ached with an intensity I couldn't bear. I stumbled toward them, my voice trembling with despair. "Why is this so amusing?" I pleaded. They looked at me, wide-eyed and speechless, as if I was the one who had shattered everything. "Please, sir, you must find a way to calm yourself," one of them pleaded.

"How can I possibly calm down?" How can you find joy when my heart is shattering, and my daughter is slipping away? My voice trembled, and the weight of my sorrow erupted into a storm of rage.

"If you don't calm yourself, we'll have to ask you to leave," another nurse said, her voice devoid of warmth. It felt surreal, like a heavy weight pressing down on my chest. My entire existence was crumbling, and they had the nerve to intimidate me. I held back my words, not out of choice, but because the pain of being forced away from my daughter in her last moments was too much to endure.

Later, as they got ready to hand her over to my ex for one final farewell, they took the blood tube from her arm. It just feels so wrong, like everything fell apart in the most painful way. Crimson flowed freely, marking my ex's dress with a haunting reminder of what once was. The sight of it—her blood—shattered me completely. My knees gave way beneath me.

And then it was finally my turn.

They placed her in my arms, her delicate form feeling so incredibly fragile, as if she might shatter at any moment. My heart raced with fear as I reached out to hold her, trembling at the thought of causing her any pain, yet deep down, I understood that this moment was everything. The oxygen tube was taken away, and I could feel her struggle through her last, heavy breaths.

The room was engulfed in a heavy silence. Her chest rose

and fell, each breath a fragile whisper, barely clinging to life. I barely managed to whisper to her, pouring out my heart, confessing my love, and expressing my deep remorse. And then, she vanished from my life. In an instant, everything changed. Her fragile form lay motionless, and the heaviness of my grief enveloped me completely.

I found myself in a secluded corner of the hospital, desperately reaching out to my family. They were completely unaware of my struggles, oblivious to the fact that I was living without a home, and they had no idea that I had a daughter who depended on me. It was as if the words were strangers, slipping from my lips, leaving a hollow ache in their wake.

"She's gone," I whispered, my voice trembling with despair.

The silence stretched endlessly on the other end, a void that echoed my despair. There's an emptiness that lingers, a silence that echoes where comfort should be. Only an unbearable silence. I hung up, engulfed by a profound sense of loneliness that I had never experienced before.

My ex was enveloped by her family, their sorrow a heavy weight that we all bore together. Yet, I found myself utterly alone. I sat in that hospital room, feeling the crushing burden of my sorrow all by myself.

I found myself trapped in a relentless loop, haunted by every moment—the call that shattered my world, the drive that felt endless, the nurses who tried to comfort, and the haunting memory of her final breaths. The void was overwhelming.

That night, I walked away from the hospital, empty and shattered, without my daughter, without a place to call home, and without a single soul to support me. I was merely a father, left with nothing but hollow arms and a heart in ruins. The world seemed to have lost all warmth, becoming a harsh and shadowy place, more unforgiving than I could have ever imagined.

The months following my daughter's departure felt like an endless haze of emptiness and sorrow, a relentless ache that consumed every moment. Time seemed to freeze, trapping me in a haunting limbo between the torment of what had transpired and the desolation of a future that felt impossible to face. The memory of my daughter's delicate form lingers, her small chest gently rising and falling for the final time in my embrace, an unbearable weight on my heart. The world continued to turn, oblivious to the pain that consumed me. It felt like an unbearable weight, crushing me from the inside.

I sought solace in the one thing that offered a fleeting escape—alcohol. What once was a casual indulgence has now turned into a haunting ritual that I can't escape from. A desperate plea for peace from the turmoil within me. A desperate attempt to fill the void that consumes me. But it just wasn't enough. It was never meant to be.

I began to blend my drinks with anything I could scrounge up. Those haunting memories linger like shadows, a painful reminder of trust shattered and innocence lost. Tablets that whispered of a realm where numbness would cradle my shattered heart, shielding me from the unbearable weight of my sorrow. And for a fleeting moment, it felt like everything was right. If only the burdens could fade away, my thoughts would dissolve into nothingness, and I might find solace in oblivion. For just a fleeting moment, I could escape the pain.

Yet, every morning, the anguish greeted me as I opened my eyes. The profound emptiness, the aching void. It felt like each sip, each tablet, only deepened the chasm within me, leaving the ache more exposed and unbearable. I felt utterly lost, unsure of how to mend the pieces of my shattered heart. I was lost in uncertainty, torn between my desires and the weight of my heartache. All I long for is the end of this unbearable suffering.

In the depths of my despair, I found myself wandering back to One Roof Youth Services once more. I felt utterly lost, with no place left to turn. I felt so lost, torn between the suffocating weight of loneliness and the unbearable presence of others. It was a cruel paradox that left me aching inside. So, I arrived there, barely holding myself together, my mind a whirlwind, my stomach in knots from the toxic blend of alcohol and drugs.

I sat there, lost in a haze, time slipping away from me, until everything changed in an instant. But in that moment, an unbearable wave of nausea crashed over me, consuming every ounce of my being. My body finally reached its breaking point, overwhelmed by the toxic burden I had been inflicting upon it for weeks, and I collapsed right there in the heart of the office.

The world around me blurred into a haze as I heaved, my insides twisting painfully, spilling my anguish onto the floor. The sound was unbearable, but the true agony lay in the expressions of the staff and the others present in the room. Utter despair. Such deep sorrow.

I recall a staff member approaching me, attempting to engage in conversation, but her words were lost to me. It felt as though I was drowning, lost in a world where everything was muffled and distant. Her words felt like whispers lost in the void, her voice a haunting echo fading away. All I could think about was how desperately I longed to just fade into nothingness.

"Do you want help?" she asked, her voice trembling with unspoken pain.

I'm lost and in need of support. It was a word that echoed in my mind, a haunting reminder of something I had never truly embraced. No amount of help could ever fill the void left by my daughter's absence. It was never going to heal the deep ache within me.

I just couldn't believe it. "I can't." "Please, just go away."

I felt an overwhelming urge to let out a cry that echoed the depths of my despair. I longed to express the depth of my pain, the overwhelming desire to vanish from this world. But I just couldn't. It felt as if my spirit had surrendered, utterly exhausted from the endless struggle.

I went through the motions of trying to piece myself back together, of uttering apologies to everyone for the chaos I had created, but it all felt so empty. Void. The anguish within me felt insurmountable, rendering any words of remorse utterly meaningless.

That night, I drowned my sorrows in more drinks. And so much more. No matter how hard I fought, the memories and the heartache clung to me like shadows, refusing to let go. No matter how much effort I put in, I only sank further into despair. The alcohol became more than just an escape; it turned into a cruel form of self-punishment. I feel like I have let my daughter down in the most profound way. I feel like I've let myself down in the most profound way. I was never meant to experience any joy.

And so, I drank to escape, to dull the ache, the regret, and the heartache that had woven itself into the very fabric of my being. I turned to the bottle, hoping to silence the haunting dreams and the endless flow of tears that just wouldn't cease. I turned to drinking, believing it was the sole escape from the overwhelming ache that consumed me.

Yet, even through the fog of my intoxication, a painful truth lingered—I understood it would never be enough. It will never be enough. The alcohol would fade, leaving me alone with the pain, as piercing and fresh as the moment I first encountered it.

I found myself caught in a painful struggle, feeling as though I was trapped in a world where existence felt unbearable, yet the thought of leaving it all behind filled me with dread. I found myself ensnared, confined within the walls of my own despair. And despite the deep shame that consumed me, I found myself unable to break free. I felt utterly lost, trapped in a whirlwind of despair, unable to find a way out.

In those moments, I felt utterly invisible, as if my very existence had faded away. Nothing at all. I feel like a mere shadow of who I once was. A father who had let everyone down. A soul lost in an ocean of sorrow, desperately searching for a glimmer of hope to rise again.

6

Finding A Glimmer of Hope

I can't pinpoint the moment I fell into despair, but I vividly recall the day everything began to shift. Perhaps it wasn't the absolute lowest point, but it certainly felt that way. After all the drinking, the numbness, the relentless self-loathing—I felt utterly empty. Nowhere to turn, no hope left to cling to. I found myself trapped, suffocating in the depths of my despair, accompanied only by the haunting presence of my daughter, a bittersweet reminder of my shattered heart.

But then, everything shattered in an instant. The call came, shattering everything I thought I knew. For months, I felt lost, drifting from one shelter to another, desperately seeking a place to belong, only to find myself on different couches, never truly at home. One Roof Youth Services—the place I had once turned to for solace, the roofies, was a lifeline that increasingly felt like a heavy weight on my heart. The kindness of the people felt like a fleeting light in an overwhelming, chaotic storm that left me feeling lost and shattered. It felt like an endless cycle of anguish. Overdoses were occurring with such frequency that it felt like a haunting reality we had to endure. It felt impossible to escape that endless loop.

The roofies drifted in and out of the office, lost and searching, forever chasing their next escape or grappling with the haunting remnants of their last encounter. The haunting images of those lost souls linger in my mind, their bodies sprawled, lifeless and still, as time drags on in agonizing silence, waiting for a voice to break the despair and summon aid. The paramedics arrived, the Narcan in their hands, and the overwhelming dread of realizing how close we were to losing everything consumed us. It served as an unending reminder of the delicate state of our existence. Amidst the overwhelming shadows, a flicker of hope emerged, offering a glimpse of something that felt so distant yet so desperately needed.

Next Steps Housing (NSH)—a transitional housing program that welcomed souls like mine, those who had endured unimaginable pain, and offered a glimmer of hope to start anew. In the beginning, it felt impossible to accept. I believed it was merely another shattered promise, yet another flicker of hope that would lead to disappointment. But then they reached out to me. They told me I was accepted.

I'll always remember the overwhelming surge of feelings that engulfed me. A piece of my soul was consumed by anger and bitterness, convinced that I was unworthy of any kindness or support. Yet, buried deep within me—fragile, nearly undetectable—there flickered a faint glimmer of hope. For the first time in what feels like an eternity, I finally found something to cling to.

I found myself in the NSH facility, a place that was meant to provide some semblance of stability and a glimmer of hope for the future. Yet, even within this so-called "safe" space, it turned out to be far more complicated than I ever imagined. The haunting presence of addiction, violence, and trauma loomed around me, suffocating every breath I took. The roofies had haunted me.

People drifted in and out of my life, some barely lasting a few weeks before succumbing to their demons, their lifeless forms scattered across the hallways, in beds, on couches. It served as an unyielding reminder of the swift descent we could face, how delicate existence truly is. It felt like a cruel twist of fate, witnessing it unfold at One Roof, and now, here it was again, tearing at my heart.

It was heartbreaking to see friends I had cherished for so long stumble once again into the same painful patterns. The faces I once shared laughter and tears with now lay motionless, their spirits momentarily revived by Narcan, only to slip back into the same heartbreaking cycle the next day.

Individuals who had been worn down to their very core, perpetually fraught with tension, perpetually on the brink of breaking down. Sometimes, it felt as if I were treading on shards of glass, paralyzed by the fear of making a single misstep, overwhelmed by the dread of opening my heart to anyone. Yet, the most unbearable aspect was the overwhelming guilt. Even with a roof over my head, a supposed safe haven, an overwhelming sense of not belonging clung to me like a shadow, refusing to let go. It felt as if I was witnessing everything, I held dear fall apart, and yet I was utterly powerless to intervene.

There were days when the weight of the world kept me trapped beneath the sheets, unable to face another moment. I felt utterly shattered, overwhelmed by the crushing burden of all that was gone, all the mistakes I had made, and the things I could never take back. The alcohol and the drugs lingered like shadows, constantly murmuring in the depths of my thoughts. But now, I find myself faced with a choice that weighs heavily on my heart. I'm trapped in this endless loop, torn between surrendering to the pain or mustering the strength to resist.

It felt unbearable. It was always going to be a struggle. Yet in the stillness, my heart ached for my daughter. I reflected on the deep ache within me, the dreams I had envisioned, and the uncertain future that seemed so far out of reach, leaving me questioning my worthiness. And I understood that I had to keep going, even though every step felt like a weight on my heart. For her, my heart aches endlessly. For me, it feels like a heavy weight that I can't shake off, a constant reminder of what once was. The ache is unbearable, and every moment is a struggle to find solace in a world that feels so empty without you.

But every step forward felt like it was accompanied by a crushing weight of a hundred steps back. I was left in a void, searching for clarity that never came. There were no promises to hold onto. All I had was a fragile glimmer of hope that perhaps, just perhaps, I could escape the suffocating shadows that surrounded me.

There was a day, not long after I moved into Next Steps Housing, when the weight of the world felt unbearable once more. The agony of losing my daughter, the crushing burden of addiction, the haunting solitude and sense of being forsaken—it all overwhelmed me in an instant. I felt utterly lost, as if I had exhausted every possibility, and for the first time in ages, I was engulfed in a darkness that seemed to have no escape. It seemed as though all hope had vanished, leaving me with an unbearable emptiness that made it impossible to find a reason to carry on. The thought of finding a way out felt like the sole choice, the only release from the overwhelming shadows that had enveloped me for what felt like an eternity.

I was sitting in my room, overwhelmed by the relentless thoughts that had been haunting me for weeks. The walls seemed to suffocate me, tightening their grip with every breath I took. My heart ached, burdened by a sorrow that felt insurmountable. My mind was a fog, my chest felt heavy, and in that instant, surrender seemed like the only option.

But just as I thought I had finally found my way, something utterly unforeseen shattered everything. My phone buzzed, and my heart sank. It was a message from the sister missionaries at the LDS church, and it felt like a bittersweet reminder of everything that once was. It feels like an eternity since I last heard their voice. They were a gentle light in my darkest moments, providing warmth and understanding when I felt utterly lost. Yet, this message, this fragile whisper of hope, shattered the silence and altered my world forever.

They reached out, asking how I was doing, trying to remind me that I wasn't alone, but the weight of their words felt like a fragile thread barely holding me together. It was a small gesture, yet it felt like a fragile thread of hope amidst the chaos, desperately clinging to me as I struggled to stay afloat.

I felt utterly lost, overwhelmed by the weight of it all. I felt so lost and alone, unable to find faith in anything, especially not in God. I have never experienced that kind of love. I have spent my life surrounded by anguish, by deceit, by heartache. I had come to depend solely on myself, to place my trust in no one, particularly not in some unseen, intangible force that felt so distant and unreachable. To me, God felt like an enigma, a remote presence that seemed indifferent to the struggles of someone like me. The weight of my suffering felt unbearable, and the shattered pieces of my heart left me unable to trust in anything anymore.

But this message, it awakened a deep ache within me. For the first time in what feels like an eternity, I caught a fleeting glimpse of something that wasn't just overwhelming sorrow. I was drawn in, compelled to listen, as if this fleeting moment held the weight of everything I had lost.

I found myself sitting with the missionaries once more, desperately seeking answers, yearning to understand the chaos swirling within me. Gradually, piece by piece, I found myself releasing the heavy weight of my doubts. I began to think that perhaps there was something beyond my own existence, something far more profound. The transformation didn't happen in a single moment. I didn't just accept everything they said without question. But the more I searched for meaning, the more I felt an overwhelming ache for something greater than myself. In the midst of my turmoil, there were fleeting moments of tranquility—soft murmurs that soothed my aching heart, a love that felt so profound yet so painfully out of reach.

And then, one day, I found myself at a crossroads, burdened by the weight of my choices. I had plans to be baptized.

The day of my baptism felt like a dream, a moment that should have been filled with joy, yet it left me feeling hollow and lost. It was a day I never imagined would arrive, a day I never believed I could summon the strength to confront. As I stood in that water, ready to take the plunge, I felt the weight of my past pressing down on me—the pain, the heartbreak, the self-doubt—overwhelming and relentless, yet somehow beginning to wash away. I stood there, trembling at the brink of an unfamiliar reality, a reality I had never dared to imagine could exist.

As I emerged from the water, a fleeting sense of weightlessness washed over me, but it was quickly overshadowed by the heaviness in my heart. It was as if a glimmer of hope had been offered to me, a moment where I believed that something divine had reached into my existence. The weight I had borne for what felt like an eternity—of guilt, of shame, of anger—was gradually starting to fade away. After what felt like an eternity, I finally found a moment to breathe. I started to place my trust in God, not because everything was clear, but because deep down, I felt his presence through all the pain and uncertainty. Even in my darkest moments, when His presence felt so distant and my trust wavered, He was there, quietly leading me through the depths of my suffering.

It felt so ordinary, so painfully real. It felt like a never-ending struggle. There are still moments when the shadows loom, ready to engulf me once more. But now, I clung to a fragile thread—something that offered a flicker of hope when the weight of despair felt unbearable. I once held onto a belief, not in the concept of God, but in the warmth of His love that tried to mend the deep void within me. I had come to understand that the enigma of God was not a source of dread, but rather a profound truth to hold close to my heart. There were countless questions swirling in my mind, so many things that felt impossibly out of reach. Yet, I had tried to trust, to release my grip, to convince myself that I belonged to something greater, even when the entire scene remained hidden from my view.

And from that moment on, everything started to unravel. Not all at once, but piece by piece, painfully, as if each moment stretches the heart just a little more. God had raised me from the depths in ways I could never have fathomed. In the tiniest fragments of time, I sensed Him—like the gentle compassion of the sun on my face, breaking through the suffocating shadows that had consumed me, and the fragile tranquility that finally settled in my heart after an endless storm of despair. It felt like a cruel twist of fate, and it shattered my heart.

For the first time in my life, I felt a connection, as if the weight of solitude had finally lifted, if only for a moment. Perhaps, there was a light within me amongst this endless darkness.

7

Building Something Bigger

After my baptism, I felt an overwhelming darkness that surrounded me. It wasn't merely about seeking faith; it was about discovering a path, a way to pour my anguish and the weight of my experiences into something meaningful. Deep down, I realized that my existence could no longer unfold in the same heart-wrenching manner it always had. There had to be something beyond this pain—a way to not just endure but to leave a mark on the world. That's when the fragile beginnings of my entrepreneurial journey started to emerge, filled with uncertainty and longing.

I was lost in my ignorance of business, yet deep down, I felt an aching desire to create change. I had come across Life Leadership, a company that claims to be founded on the ideals of personal growth and leadership, but it feels like a distant hope now. When I first signed up, I felt a flicker of hope, but deep down, I was lost and unsure of what this program would bring into my life. It was about nurturing your own soul to uplift others—a sentiment that struck a profound chord within me. After all that I have endured, I came to understand that leadership transcends power or control; it is truly about serving, about elevating others in their darkest moments.

In those early months, I lost myself in their teachings, desperately seeking solace in every word. I clung to audio programs, and consumed books about success, mindset, and resilience. It was never truly easy. There were countless moments when I questioned my worth, feeling lost and unsure if I could ever create something that truly mattered. Yet, I found myself moving forward, and slowly, I started to piece together the fragile beauty of connection. Life Leadership felt like more than just personal development; it was a fragile hope for a community of souls yearning to make a difference in a world that often feels so heavy and unforgiving.

In this vast network, I found souls who saw something in me, even when I was lost in my own doubts and shadows. The deep yearning I have to help others, and they urged me to dream beyond the confines of my shattered heart. That's when I understood that my path wasn't merely about piecing my life back together—it was about transforming my pain into something that could touch and alter the lives of others.

This revelation pushed me to take a leap of faith, pouring my heart into nurturing 'Hearts Healing Humanity', the charity I had founded. The thought had lingered in the shadows, quietly haunting me, but now it seems like the moment has arrived to surrender completely. It began with just a few volunteers and a fragile hope to reach out to those who needed it most. I longed to become the very person I had yearned for in my most despairing times. I longed to provide a glimmer of hope, a comforting hand to grasp, and a way to move ahead for those who seemed utterly lost.

Running 'Hearts Healing Humanity' felt like an insurmountable struggle. There were days when the weight of the world pressed down on me, leaving me gasping for breath amidst the endless cries for help. The stories I heard—the pain, the struggles—echoed my own journey, and at times, it felt impossible to detach myself from the work. Yet, each time I witnessed someone bravely taking their first steps toward a brighter future, it pierced my heart, reminding me of the dreams I once held so dearly.

I gave my all to the charity, leaving nothing behind. I discovered the painful art of crafting grant proposals, the heart-wrenching experience of reaching out to local businesses, and the bittersweet struggle of uniting communities for a cause that feels so far away. In my quest to make a difference, I reached out to food banks, housing organizations, and various nonprofits, hoping to create a ripple of change that could ease the burden of those in need. It was an incredibly challenging journey, yet I clung to the hope that this was my true calling. Every success, no matter how small, felt like a bittersweet victory—not just for the people we helped, but for me, too, as I grappled with the weight of my own heartache.

The connections I once began to forge through Life Leadership now feel like a distant memory, leaving an ache that lingers in my heart. These were souls who truly grasped the essence of dreaming big, who bravely confronted challenges, and who persevered even when everything seemed stacked against them. They were once my guiding lights, my partners in creation, and the closest of companions. They showed me how to envision a future filled with hope, how to transform every setback into a chance for growth, and how to push through the darkness, even when the way ahead felt impossibly uncertain.

As Hearts Healing Humanity blossomed, I felt myself unraveling. The charity transformed into something far deeper than a mere project; it embodied all the lessons I had gathered about enduring pain, clinging to hope, and the fragile strength found within a community. It became a desperate attempt to transform my anguish into something meaningful, to somehow offer something back that acknowledged the battles I had fought through.

As I reflect on my past, I can't help but feel the weight of every moment that brought me to this painful place. The shadows I have faced, the painful lessons that have scarred me, and the souls I have crossed paths with—each moment has carved me into the fragile being I am now, desperately trying to carry out this mission. And even though there were still challenges looming in the distance, a spark ignited me, a feeling I thought I had lost forever. For the first time, I was trying to create something meaningful, something that might endure beyond my own existence, something that could bring a shimmer of light that was brought into the darkness. This was merely the start, and I was hopeful to discover where this journey might lead me.

I started to reveal my story, piece by piece, in the quiet corners of small gatherings: community meetings, workshops, and events held by other nonprofits, where the weight of my words felt both heavy and necessary. Every moment, I felt the weight of my words crushing those around me. I wasn't merely sharing my experiences—I was clinging to the fragile thread of hope, a whisper that even in the depths of despair, there might still be a path ahead. People would approach me afterward, their eyes glistening with tears, expressing how deeply they connected with my journey or how my words had ignited a flicker of hope within them to persevere. It was a moment that shattered me, yet it deepened my conviction that my voice, though fragile, could still be a beacon for change.

As I wrapped up my initial speaking engagements, a deep longing stirred within me, a yearning for something greater, something more profound. Motivational speaking became more than just sharing my story; it transformed into a desperate plea to convey the fragile essence of resilience and empowerment that I had clung to in the darkest moments of my life. I started to reach out to schools, organizations, and even local businesses, desperately trying to share my story about overcoming adversity, the strength of community, and the hope that we can all make a difference. People were eager to listen to my story of how I transformed my life from the depths of homelessness into a beacon of prosperity and how I discovered faith and a sense of purpose even when everything felt lost and broken.

In that moment, I felt overwhelmed, carrying a weight that seemed unbearable. I had found the courage to re-enroll in university, clinging to the hope of finally completing my degree. Juggling school, Hearts Healing Humanity, and my emerging career as a speaker felt like an insurmountable challenge, leaving me overwhelmed and lost. There were days when I felt utterly shattered, as if I was being pulled apart and I didn't know how I could possibly carry on. Yet, in the depths of my despair, when the thought of surrender loomed large, a flicker of the reasons that ignited my journey would surface, reminding me of the light that once shone so brightly. Education was once a cherished dream of mine—a reminder to unlock doors, gather the knowledge and skills I desperately needed to piece together a better life for myself and those I cared about.

As my speaking career blossomed, my dreams of entrepreneurship began to swell, yet they felt so distant and unattainable. 'Hearts Healing Humanity' continued to thrive, lost in thoughts about how to create a lasting impact amidst the overwhelming weight of my emotions. I started to create new social enterprises, each one deeply connected to the values that had sustained me during my most painful moments. In every moment, I poured my heart into helping others find a place to call home, nurturing their dreams, and seeking out new paths to uplift those who felt lost. My mind was always racing with ideas, yet the weight of it all felt so heavy.

I found myself turning my attention to those around me—trying to guide others, sharing the fragments of wisdom I had gathered, and supporting them as they took their hesitant first steps toward a brighter tomorrow. It was painfully bittersweet to witness others thrive, to feel the weight of knowing I had a fleeting role in their journey. In the faces of those I worked alongside, I found reflections of myself—echoes of the struggles, shadows of the fears, and the fragile light of their dreams. I wished for them to understand that they, too, could rise above the darkest of struggles.

Motivational speaking transformed into something far deeper than a mere career; it evolved into a heartfelt mission that resonates with the very core of my being. Standing on stage, gazing out at a sea of faces yearning for hope, I was overwhelmed by a profound sense of purpose that pierced through my heart. I wasn't merely speaking to them—I was pouring my heart out, sharing something deeply profound and vulnerable. I shared the moments that shattered my spirit and the fleeting instances that brought me a sense of completeness. I shared my struggles with heartache, the emptiness of loss, the flicker of hope, and the unwavering wish that someday, somehow, things might improve.

One of the most poignant moments of my speaking career unfolded when a member of the audience approached me after my talk, their eyes filled with unshed tears, and said, "I was on the brink of surrender, but your story gave me hope." It served as a haunting reminder of the reasons I clung to hope, even when every step felt unbearable. Every person I reached felt like a fleeting moment of triumph, each life I touched a bittersweet reminder of what once was, urging me to keep speaking, building, and growing despite the weight of my heart.

By the end of that year, I had achieved things that felt like distant dreams, now hauntingly bittersweet. I poured my heart into a charity that was transforming lives, started businesses that were truly impactful, and opened up my soul to thousands, sharing my story with them. I thought I had finally achieved something meaningful, showing myself and the world that I could overcome every challenge in my path. And through it all, I was desperately clinging to a purpose and faith that barely held me together in the darkest of times.

8

The Lessons I Learned

As I look back on my journey, I realize that every challenge, every moment of joy, and each relationship I built led me to a profound understanding: love is truly what matters most. Embracing love for others, cherishing life, and, most importantly, nurturing love for ourselves.

Being autistic is an experience that often eludes the understanding of many. I have my own unique perspective. The lessons that have shaped who I am go beyond merely surviving difficult moments; they revolve around transformation and welcoming love, even in the face of adversity and pain.

As someone on the autism spectrum, I've always experienced the world through a unique perspective marked by deep sensitivity and sharp observation. Life has certainly had its challenges. On the contrary, it's been filled with moments where I've felt out of place, alone, and weighed down.

Through these struggles, I've found a deep sense of clarity. I notice beauty in places that others might miss, and I connect with people and environments in ways that go beyond what words can convey.

This perspective on life has shown me that love goes beyond just feeling; it's about actively engaging with and embracing both others and ourselves. It's about embracing kindness even in tough times, letting go when it seems unthinkable, and treating ourselves with care when we falter. It's a decision we embrace repeatedly, even when it seems like everything around us is opposing our path.

Each challenge I've encountered has deepened my understanding of this truth. Being autistic has allowed me to perceive the true nature of things, recognizing that love transcends grand gestures and flawless moments. It's in the steady determination, the little gestures of goodwill, and the bravery to continue on, even when life seems too much to bear.

Throughout this journey, I've come to value the moments of connection and joy that arise from fully embracing my true self. I've realized that my differences are not shortcomings but valuable assets. They have influenced me to appreciate sincerity, to pursue meaningful connections in every exchange, and to hold the belief that love is fundamentally what truly counts.

If there's one thing, I hope others take away from my story, it's this: Our differences shape our identities, and by embracing them—and the love that connects us all—we discover our greatest strength.

These are the insights that life and love have shared with me:

1. Life Is More Than Material Possessions—It's About Our Way of Life

In life, we enter this world with nothing, and we depart in the same manner. What really counts is the way we live our lives—how we interact with others, how we stand by our principles, and the love we share and embrace. What truly defines us isn't the things we own or the awards we collect; it's the acts of kindness we show, the honesty in our decisions, and the connections we build with others. Embracing each other, with all our imperfections and unique traits, creates a legacy that holds far greater significance than any material possession.

2. Pain Can't Be Wiped Away, but It Can Be Changed

Pain is always there—it doesn't go away, no matter how much we hope it will. I've come to realize that pain doesn't have to break us; rather, it can serve as the inspiration for something truly beautiful. When we transform our pain into love—when we decide to forgive, to heal, and to contribute—we reshape our destiny. Two wrongs don't create a right outcome. Real revenge isn't about anger or getting back at someone; it's about embracing love and not allowing the hurt someone inflicted to shape who we are. Transforming darkness into light is the ultimate triumph.

3. True Happiness Is Found Within

For a long time, I looked for happiness in others, in possessions, and in situations. I sought validation, acceptance, and joy from others, but I often found disappointment instead. I came to understand that true happiness comes from within. It's really about our inner perspective and how we view ourselves and our experiences. Critics, obstacles, and difficulties will always be part of life, but when we cease depending on external validation and begin to discover our own inner joy, we become resilient. True happiness that comes from loving yourself is something that can never be lost.

4. At the Heart of All Our Challenges Lies a Deficit of Self-Love

Every challenge I encountered—from unhealthy relationships to harmful habits—originated from a single core problem: I lacked self-love. When we lack self-love, we settle for less than what we truly deserve, seek validation in ways that aren't beneficial, and permit others to mistreat us. Self-love goes beyond affirmations and pampering; it involves acknowledging our value, establishing boundaries, and having faith that we are worthy of good things. When we embrace who we are, we can genuinely extend that love to others and live our truth.

5. Love Is the Most Powerful Energy in Existence

Love goes beyond mere emotion; it's about taking action, making choices, and harnessing a powerful force that can achieve the impossible. It's about how we are there for others, even when it's challenging. Forgiveness is found in the grace we extend, even when it's not warranted. It's the hope we hold onto, even when everything around us seems dark. Love can mend wounds, connect people, and foster something enduring and meaningful.

6. Appreciation Welcomes Love

Gratitude allows us to appreciate the beauty in life, even when faced with challenges. It's simple to dwell on our shortcomings or what's missing, but embracing gratitude allows us to see things differently. Gratitude involves acknowledging pain while also recognizing the blessings that can emerge from it. When we express gratitude for the lessons, the connections, and even the challenges, we open ourselves up to love and abundance in our lives.

7. Love Is the Legacy We Make

When everything is said and done, what do we truly leave behind? It's not about material things; it's the love we've experienced together. It's the connections we've made and the compassion we've shared. Love is the one thing that flourishes when shared, and it's what endures when all else diminishes. When we embrace love as our core value, we create a lasting impact that transcends our time here.

8. Pay Attention and Strive for Clarity

One of the most challenging lessons I learned was the significance of truly listening—not only to those around me but also to the essence of life itself. Too frequently, we hurry to reply, to explain, to validate our own perspectives. True growth starts when we take a moment to pause, listen, and genuinely seek to understand the lessons that life presents to us. Life is not about proving a point; it's about embracing the insights that arise from a place of humility and patience. Every experience, no matter how difficult, offers us valuable lessons if we are open to understanding them.

These lessons were more than just realizations; they were profound awakenings that transformed my identity and influenced my way of living. They've empowered me to heal, to evolve, and to continue progressing with intention.

When I lost my daughter, everything I understood fell apart. In the silence that came after, I found myself confronting the questions that linger for everyone when faced with loss: What does it all mean? What's the significance of this? For a long time, I found myself preoccupied with concerns about finances, seeking security, and attempting to define my value based on my accomplishments or possessions. But as I stood in the aftermath of her passing, none of those things seemed significant anymore. The fear of homelessness and the stress of financial insecurity were indeed significant, but they faded when compared to the profound, irreplaceable impact of losing her.

In those moments, I came to a deep understanding: we enter this world with nothing, and when we depart, we carry nothing away. All the money, all the belongings, and every achievement we gather in this life will ultimately remain here. The lasting effect we leave on others is what truly matters—the love we share, the kindness we express, and the values we stand by. What truly defines us isn't the possessions we gather, but the way we choose to live our lives. My daughter didn't have the opportunity to grow old, to gather wealth or accolades, but she made a lasting impression on my heart. She reminded me that the essence of life lies not in what we own, but in the moments we share.

For a long time, I was pursuing what I believed to be success. I thought that if I could simply earn enough and change my situation, everything would eventually fall into place for me. In those quiet, grief-stricken days, I came to understand that success goes beyond wealth or comfort. It's about staying true to oneself. It's about staying true to your beliefs and principles, even when external pressures encourage you to waver. It's about being present with kindness and understanding, particularly during the toughest times.

I reflected on the individuals I met during my tough times—those who showed me kindness when I had nothing to offer back. Their generosity came from a place of love, not from any desire for personal gain. The love and integrity we show truly create a lasting impact. I want to create a legacy that my daughter can cherish.

Her loss opened my eyes to a new perspective on life. It revealed the reality of what really counts. It wasn't the worry about finances that brought me down; it was the sorrow of missing out on time, love, and meaningful connections. I have decided to live in a way that truly honors her—not by pursuing superficial goals, but by embracing the values that bring real meaning to life.

Love has been my compass. It wasn't about achieving perfection—I understood I would stumble—but about working towards being someone who supports others, who hears with empathy, who offers forgiveness even when it's challenging. I started to realize that how we treat others, how we present ourselves, and how we engage with the world are the most genuine indicators of a fulfilling life.

Ultimately, life is not defined by what we leave behind. It's about the care we give to those around us and the honesty we maintain when faced with difficulties. My daughter's short stay with us here on earth showed me that the most important things in life are those that defy measurement—love, kindness, and the choices we make every single day.

This chapter of my life marked a significant change. It was no longer merely about getting by; it became a journey of embracing life with intention, passion, and a steadfast dedication to authenticity. I decided to pay tribute to her by moving ahead with love, understanding that our true essence and the way we live are what really counts in the end.

9

Pain into Purpose

Pain has always been there with me. From my earliest memories, it was always there, influencing my world in ways I never anticipated. I have witnessed the overwhelming impact directly—not only in my own experiences but also in the experiences of countless others. I've seen individuals struggle with the burden of their decisions and the pain they carry. I've lost friends to overdoses, to self-inflicted harm, to struggles they couldn't overcome. Every death has etched itself into my being, adding another scar to a heart that already bears the weight of profound loss. I understand the feeling of being trapped, and I've witnessed the outcomes of that journey.

For years, I sought ways to escape my pain. I sought solace in alcohol, believing it might help me forget the painful memories of a troubled childhood, the heartache of losing my daughter, and the burden of just trying to get by. I believed that by drinking enough, I could quiet the inner voice that insisted I wasn't enough, that echoed all my losses. Yet, regardless of how much I consumed, the pain remained, ready to greet me as soon as I sobered up. The alcohol just made things more difficult. It numbed my senses, yet it couldn't reach my soul, where the true pain resided.

In those challenging times, it felt like I was fighting a struggle that was beyond my reach. Reflecting on my journey, I realize that God has been by my side all along. He allowed me to stumble and fall, not from a place of cruelty, but from a place of love. He understood that I had to face challenges to grow into who I am now. Each challenge, every sorrow, and every instance of hopelessness was molding me, imparting the wisdom I would require to support others. God didn't provide an escape from my pain because He intended for me to learn how to change it.

I started to realize that pain was something that couldn't just be wished away, no matter how much I wanted it to be. But it didn't have to break me, either. Pain might serve as my guide. It might be the inspiration I draw upon to craft something truly significant. I came to understand that allowing my pain to shape my identity would keep me stuck indefinitely. But if I embraced it—if I transformed it into compassion, into forgiveness, into action—I could reshape the narrative.

That's when everything shifted. I let go of the urge to run from my pain and began to explore how I could embrace it.

I reflected on my mental anguish, and my mental, physical, and sexual abuse that I endured. I reflected on the people I had lost, those who didn't make it through. I reflected on my marriage and its relationships, and my daughter, whose life, though brief, was incredibly rich in significance. I reflected on the many others who were still out there, facing their own struggles, feeling as though hope was out of reach. I can't alter what has already happened, but I can decide to support others in shaping their own paths ahead.

I embraced love—not for its simplicity, but because it was the only path ahead. I decided to let go of the hurt caused by others, not out of a sense of obligation, but because clinging to anger only held me back from moving forward. I decided to share my experiences, using my struggles to reach out to those who are also in pain. In that process, I found my way to healing.

Honestly, two wrongs don't create a right. Seeking revenge won't lead to peace; it merely perpetuates the cycle of suffering. The true triumph lies in embracing love and not allowing the dark shadows to take over. Transforming your pain into light is a powerful expression of resilience.

God didn't remove my pain, but he taught me how to embrace it. He showed me that my pain was not a punishment; it was a gift. It provided me with understanding, strength, and a sense of purpose beyond my own existence. It showed me that the most powerful form of revenge comes not from anger or resentment, but from true love.

I decided to take a step forward. I decided to allow my pain to shape me, instead of letting it break me down. I decided to start shining brightly through the dark clouds both for my own sake and for those around me. I decided to reshape my karma, not by wiping away the past, but by embracing it to build a brighter future. Whenever I lend a hand to someone, or extend kindness and forgiveness, I sense a deeper connection to my own healing journey.

Suffering is always present, yet it doesn't have to shape who we are. We have the option to embrace it, transforming it into something truly beautiful. When we embrace this, we transform not just our own narratives, but also the world we inhabit. Love holds incredible strength, and through my experiences with pain, I've learned this valuable lesson.

As I was growing up, I had no understanding of what happiness truly meant. I experienced rejection, isolation, and the hurt of harsh words thrown at me on the playground or in the classroom. The kids who bullied me seemed unaware of the impact of their actions—or perhaps they were fully aware. Regardless, their words struck hard, leaving marks on my self-esteem. I can still recall the experience of entering school each day, preparing myself for the teasing, the laughter directed at me, the sense that no matter my efforts, I would never measure up. It felt like bearing a hidden hurt that remained unseen, yet everyone seemed to prod at it.

I held onto their words for quite a while. I accepted the labels they placed on me. I felt like I had no value, as if kindness and love were not meant for me. The emotions I experienced in childhood didn't just fade away; they carried into my adult life, influencing my self-perception and how I viewed the world. I looked for happiness in others, wishing that someone—anyone—might be able to fill the emptiness within me. I looked for it in possessions, believing that if I accumulated more or accomplished more, I would finally feel sufficient, and at peace. Every time I sought something outside myself for happiness, I found only disappointment.

You really can't give your all if you're running on empty. Regardless of how much love or validation you seek from others, it will always fall short if you don't recognize your own worth from within. That was a tough lesson for me to grasp, yet it turned out to be one of the most significant ones. I realized I needed to shift my focus from seeking happiness outside of myself to exploring what truly brings me joy within.

I began by facing the hurt that had been lingering within me for such a long time. I came to understand that what my bullies said reflected their own issues, not who I am. Their cruelty revealed their true nature, not mine. But the issue was, I had allowed their voices to shape my own. I took their words to heart and made them my reality. Repairing that damage took effort, but it was essential.

I started to realize that happiness isn't something you stumble upon—it's something you make for yourself. It's all about your perspective and how you perceive yourself and your journey. I let go of seeking approval from others and focused on how I communicate with myself. I shifted my attention away from what was missing and embraced gratitude for what I already possessed. I let go of the blame I placed on myself for how others treated me and began to appreciate my own worth, no matter if others acknowledged it.

The change didn't happen all at once. There were days when the deep dark demon returned, softly suggesting that I wasn't enough, that I didn't deserve happiness. But gradually, I discovered how to quiet those inner voices. I discovered the importance of recognizing my value, even in moments when it seemed like everything around me was working against me. I discovered the importance of appreciating the little moments and recognizing growth over flawlessness.

What truly stands out to me is that happiness grounded in self-love is something that can never be taken away. When you cease relying on external sources for happiness and begin to discover that joy within yourself, you become truly resilient. Critics, obstacles, and difficulties will always be present, but they diminish in strength when you have a clear understanding of yourself.

The experiences with bullies in my past influenced my early years, but they do not determine who I am today. I am the one who defines myself. Now, when I look in the mirror, I see someone who has grown beyond the mockery and humiliation of the past. I recognize a person who embodies strength, resilience, and deserves love—not due to others' opinions, but because I hold that belief within myself.

Transforming the hurt from bullying into a source of joy was a challenging journey, yet it imparted a lasting lesson: true happiness comes from within, untouched by external circumstances. Happiness is something you can create, cherish, and safeguard. When you create it from a place of self-love, it transforms into something that can never be taken away from you.

10

Lack of Self Love

For a long time, I struggled to grasp why I continued to make decisions that caused me pain. I found myself questioning why I remained in unhealthy relationships, why I sought solace in alcohol to escape my pain, and why I repeatedly placed myself in circumstances that only intensified my suffering. I found myself caught in a loop of poor choices, where each mistake seemed to lead to another. Reflecting on the past, everything comes into focus for me. Every poor choice, every moment of despair, every time I let someone treat me as if I were nothing—it all boiled down to one truth: I didn't embrace who I truly am.

In her transformative book You Can Heal Your Life, Louise Hay explores how the absence of self-love shows up in our lives. Her words resonated deeply with me the first time I read them. She mentioned that when we lack self-love, we communicate to the world that we are not deserving, and the world reflects that back to us. We settle for less than we truly deserve because we think that's all we are worth. We pursue those who are unable or unwilling to love us, believing that their approval will somehow complete what's missing within us. We often hold ourselves back, sometimes without even noticing, because we struggle to see that we are worthy of more.

She asked me to try an exercise. Looking in the mirror and telling myself, "I love who I am, just as I am." This made me feel so frustrated with myself that I wanted to punch the mirror. I felt like I had no value. I believed that to be the case. I had people who cared for me, but it was challenging to accept that love when I struggled to see my own value.

That was truly me. That was my reality. If I had really embraced who I am, I wouldn't have remained in relationships that tore me apart rather than uplifted me. I wouldn't have turned to alcohol, seeking to escape the pain that felt like a part of me. I wouldn't have repeatedly tested my limits to the point of breaking. I would never have let anyone treat me like I was insignificant, because deep down, I always knew my worth. I really had no idea. I really couldn't accept it. At some point, I came to believe that I didn't deserve love, not even from my own heart. That belief shaped the core of every choice I made. I found myself in difficult situations, seeking approval in places that didn't serve me, unable to recognize the worth and beauty within me that others often tried to highlight.

One night stands out in my memory, the first time I read Hay's book. I shut the book and sat quietly, reflecting on the decisions I had made throughout my life. The night I lost myself in a haze, wishing for the darkness to swallow me whole. The many moments I allowed the judgments of others to shape my identity, despite their harsh and unfounded remarks. The moments I looked in the mirror and saw only my shortcomings. Confronting those memories was challenging, but it led me to an important realization: I had been searching for something to fill a void within me that only I could truly address.

Self-love goes beyond simply complimenting yourself in the mirror or indulging in a nice meal. It's about reshaping the story you've been given regarding your identity and value. It's about embracing your scars—not with shame, but with kindness. It's about establishing boundaries with others, not out of selfishness, but because you appreciate yourself enough to safeguard your tranquility.

Embracing self-love has been a challenging path. It involved letting go of years filled with self-doubt and harsh inner criticism. It involved accepting my past errors and acknowledging the moments when I had fallen short of my own expectations. It was about viewing myself not by my setbacks, but by my strength to overcome them. It involved making a conscious choice each day to extend to myself the same kindness and respect that I had always offered to others, which I had often withheld from myself.

As I embraced who I truly am, everything started to shift. I no longer look for approval from those who are unable to provide it. I let go of the need to be perfect and stopped being hard on myself. I no longer let others define my value. I began to appreciate the beauty of my true self—not despite my challenges, but because of them.

Louise Hay wrote, "You've been criticizing yourself for years, and it hasn't helped." Consider embracing who you are and observe the outcome. Those words turned into a guiding principle for me. They reminded me that self-love is essential, not just something nice to have. Without it, we navigate through life, allowing others to shape our sense of worth. With it, we reclaim our power.

At the heart of all our challenges lies an absence of self-acceptance. It's at the core of our struggles, our missteps, our insecurities. Yet, it's also essential for our healing, our growth, and our joy. When we embrace who we truly are, we no longer settle for anything less than what we truly deserve. We let go of pursuing people and things that don't truly belong in our lives. We cease inflicting harm on ourselves as a way to flee from the hurt. Instead, we embrace our completeness.

If I had embraced who I truly am from the start, my journey could have taken a different direction. I'm present in this moment, and that's what truly counts. I've come to understand that self-love goes beyond merely rescuing yourself; it's about evolving into a better version of yourself. In that transformation, we discover the power to embrace our true selves, to love deeply, and to build a life that showcases the beauty of our genuine essence.

When I began to genuinely love others, everything started to change—not only within myself, but also in how people perceived me. For a long time, I found myself trapped in a cycle of hurt and self-defense, pushing people away and hiding my true feelings behind anger or apathy. As I embraced self-love, I realized that love isn't something to keep to myself or hold back—it's meant to be shared openly, without fear or conditions.

Initially, it was quite challenging. Embracing love involves releasing past grievances and opting for forgiveness. It involved recognizing others not as challenges or barriers, but as individuals with their own narratives, hardships, and emotions. It involved swapping out judgment for understanding and embracing the art of listening, even in moments of disagreement. When I decided to engage with others from a place of love rather than suspicion or defensiveness, I noticed something truly remarkable: people's perceptions of me began to shift.

I once felt that others perceived me as a mystery—difficult to understand, challenging to trust, and perhaps even intimidating to engage with. But when I started to express my love freely, they noticed a change. They recognized a person who truly cared, someone ready to be there for them during their toughest times. I began to create connections where barriers had previously existed. Those who had maintained their distance started to come nearer, not due to any request from me, but because love fostered an environment where they felt secure.

This transformation had a deep impact. I witnessed individuals share their true selves in ways they hadn't done previously. People who were once strangers became friends, and past hurts were mended through sincere and meaningful conversations. Love emerged as a light—one that attracted others, not due to its perfection, but because of its authenticity.

I will always remember the moment when someone shared with me how my love impacted their life. A friend who had been battling their own challenges, someone I had opened up to wholeheartedly, without any expectation of reciprocity. They shared with me that my kindness had inspired hope within them, and that my faith in them had encouraged them to believe in themselves. That moment transformed me. It opened my eyes to the fact that love is an incredible force—not only for helping others, but also for our own healing.

As I kept loving others, I noticed how this energy could

spread, bringing about change in ways I never thought possible. Love melted tough exteriors and united individuals who may have never met otherwise. It fostered relationships where there was previously separation, and it ignited optimism in areas that had seen despair.

This was about simple truths and real moments. It was in the small gestures: a thoughtful word to uplift someone struggling, a patient ear for those who felt overlooked, a smile that reassured someone they mattered. I've come to realize that love isn't about how big it is, but rather how true it is.

People began to see me differently because they recognized the sincerity of my love. It was never about personal gain or expecting anything in return. It was about recognizing the human experience in others and making the choice to be present for them, even when it was challenging or uneasy. This decision to love—genuinely love—sparked a wave of inspiration, encouraging others to follow suit.

Throughout this journey, I've discovered that love is the most powerful force in the universe, as it transforms everything it encounters. It mends wounds that appear irreparable. It connects gaps that appear impossible to cross. It changes not only those we care about but also the one who is giving that love.

Showing love to others can sometimes be challenging. It

takes openness, bravery, and the readiness to face the possibility of pain. However, the benefits are beyond measure. Choosing love allows us to build a world that shines with warmth, compassion, and deeper connections. By being a source of light for others in their moments of darkness, we also find clarity and direction for ourselves.

Love goes beyond mere emotion; it's a decision we make. Every day, I choose this path, and it has truly changed my life. As I move forward on this journey, I'm reminded of the amazing ability of love to bring about change, to heal, and to bring people together. It truly stands as the most beautiful and lasting legacy we can offer to the world.

Gratitude holds immense power. I didn't always grasp its real significance, however. For years, I moved through life focused on what I lacked—what was absent—constantly measuring my journey against those around me. I concentrated on the challenges, the setbacks, and the heartache. I convinced myself that happiness would come only after I had solved all my problems and reached my dreams. However, that's not how life operates.

The pivotal moment arrived when I found myself engulfed in profound despair, seeking a path forward. I have faced a lot—bullying, loss, addiction, and the constant struggle within my own thoughts. I attempted to fill that void with all sorts of things—money, belongings, distractions—but nothing truly resonated. I found that when I turned my gaze inward, exploring the depths of my own being, a new perspective began to unfold. I started a straightforward list of the things I appreciate. Initially, it seemed a bit unnatural and uncomfortable. I didn't have a clear view, but I knew I needed to take that first step.

It was the little things that truly transformed me. It was the small details—the moments I had ignored or failed to appreciate. The gentle touch of the morning sun on my skin, the soothing embrace of a beloved song, the unwavering support from friends who stood by me during tough times. These small moments, which felt trivial in the moment, began to accumulate, and a shift started to unfold.

As I began to embrace gratitude, I noticed a gentle change in my heart. The things I had once resented—the struggles, the pain—began to reveal their purpose. I didn't need to flee from or fight against them. They were experiences that taught valuable lessons, offered chances for personal growth, and helped in developing resilience. As I reflected on my life with a sense of appreciation, I recognized the abundance of gifts I had received. I was presented with an opportunity to evolve, to gain knowledge, and above all, to embrace love.

Feeling thankful revealed love to me in ways I never anticipated. As I embraced gratitude for my life, just as it was, I started to connect with others in a way I had never experienced before. I began to truly value the individuals who stood by me, even during my challenging moments. I began to recognize their true selves—imperfect, lovely, and deeply human—and my love for them grew unconditional. Gratitude opened my eyes to the truth that love is not about being flawless; it's about embracing one another.

I discovered that expressing gratitude deepened my feelings of love, not only for those around me but also for myself. I came to understand that I had been incredibly hard on myself for quite a while. When I opened my eyes to the good, the progress, and the lessons in my life, I began to see myself as whole. I began to see myself as deserving of love and grace.

Gratitude shifted my perspective from what was missing to a deep appreciation for what I already possessed. It completely shifted my viewpoint and helped me see that even during the toughest times, there was always something to appreciate. In those little moments, often overlooked, I discovered the true beauty of life. Gratitude not only uplifted my spirits—it connected me more deeply with others and, ultimately, with my own self.

When I embraced gratitude, I found that love started to flow into my life in wonderful ways. It's not about love that depends on situations; it's about the love we decide to embrace regardless of the challenges. Gratitude is the key—it unlocks the path to love by transforming our energy. When we concentrate on what we possess rather than what we lack, we naturally become more giving towards ourselves and those around us. We grow in patience, understanding, and our capacity to forgive.

Reaching this point has been quite a journey. There were days when I struggled to find gratitude, when the burdens of life felt overwhelming. Yet, in those moments, I made it a point to identify at least one thing to appreciate. And gradually, it came together. My heart expanded. My affection for others deepened. I developed a deeper appreciation for who I am.

Gratitude isn't merely a way to boost our mood; it's a meaningful practice that influences our lives in profound ways. Starting with gratitude allows us to transform the world we live in. By embracing love, we create a space for others to experience it as well. Gratitude is a straightforward yet deep approach to change how we see things and welcome more love into our lives. It serves as the essential element that opens the way, guiding us toward a life rich in connection, compassion, and joy.

11

Legacy

We come into this world with nothing and we leave this world with nothing. When our journey here concludes, we depart in the same way. At first glance, it might appear to be a somber notion—the belief that all the material possessions, the accolades, and the wealth we gather during our lives won't accompany us when we depart. As I think about this truth, I come to see it as the most liberating realization I've ever experienced. When we remove all the material things and distractions from our lives, what truly matters is the core of our being—the love we shared, the feelings we inspired in others, and the influence we had on those in our lives. Love is the only thing that lasts forever.

As I reflect on my life, I recognize the moments that truly shape who I am—not through possessions or accomplishments, but through the decisions I've taken and the impact those decisions have had on others. There was a time when I believed I needed to become someone important in this world—someone with money, fame, and achievements. I believed those things would give me value, would show that I truly count. Over the years, I've come to realize that everything else is insignificant if it's not rooted in love.

With each interaction, we create a connection that matters. It's a lasting experience that goes beyond the surface. We are building something meaningful, one choice at a time. When we extend kindness to those in need, advocate for justice, or offer compassion in difficult times, we create a lasting impact on the world around us. Every act of love creates waves, influencing lives in ways we might never completely grasp.

I once viewed legacy as something tangible I could pass on—perhaps some money, a business, or an inheritance of some kind. I've come to understand that the real legacy we create is the love we share. The impact we have on others, the feelings we evoke, and how we choose to spend our time to improve the world—this is what truly defines our legacy. That's what outlasts us.

Every choice we make allows us to share a part of ourselves with others. A simple gesture, a supportive action, or a shared moment of empathy can profoundly impact the course of someone's life. That individual will, in their own way, connect with others in ways that might go unnoticed. It's similar to tossing a pebble into a pond—the ripples spread far and wide, often unnoticed, yet they exist. The energy we share with the world, be it uplifting or challenging, sends out waves that linger well beyond our time here.

I realize that all my experiences—the losses, the heartaches, the challenges—were all part of something greater. I've come to realize that my struggles have purpose and meaning. I was here to learn, to grow, and to share those lessons with others. The love I share now comes from a place of deep empathy, compassion, and understanding, not just joy. I understand the feeling of hitting rock bottom. I understand the experience of feeling insignificant, isolated, and shattered. But I also understand the experience of emerging from that darkness and connecting with others who are facing their own challenges.

The love I share today is shaped by my experiences, and I offer it openly because I understand its ability to bring healing. I've witnessed the incredible impact that kindness and understanding can have on someone's life. A simple act of love can truly create a ripple that transforms everything. I want to be remembered for the love I've given, not for the possessions I've gathered.

I've come to understand that love goes beyond mere feelings; it's a decision we make. We embrace love, we embrace forgiveness, we embrace compassion, even when it's challenging. These choices shape the core of our legacy. We might not immediately notice the effects of what we do, but eventually, when we're no longer here, the people we've influenced will hold our love in their hearts. It will be shared and will keep expanding, even when we're not around anymore.

For me, this embodies the essence of creating a lasting legacy. It's not about what we leave behind; it's about embracing the present and truly experiencing life as it unfolds. It's about choosing from a place of love rather than letting fear guide you. It's about being there for others, even when it's tough. It's all about sharing kindness, joy, and compassion in every step we take. It's about understanding that love isn't only what we offer; it's also what we welcome back, forming a beautiful cycle that can endure through the years.

I've come to realize that the love I've given to others is what truly counts. It is the one thing that will live on, long after everything else fades away. Love is what we carry forward, and it's the essence that gives our lives real significance.

In January 2024, I experienced the loss of someone incredibly significant to me—my best friend, Zack who passed away at 24 years of age from an overdose inside a Tim Hortons local in Waterloo. Zack was a person who radiated a distinct vibe, someone brimming with potential. Life felt like an ongoing battle for him, with decisions that appeared to lead him further from the tranquility he desired. At his funeral, his family shared memories of him as a wonderful kid—full of heart, yet someone who often didn't pay attention. They genuinely attempted to assist him. They attempted to lead him, to illuminate the way forward, yet he found it difficult to listen to their voices. And in the end, that brought him to a point of no return. It shattered me.

At the funeral, as I stood there surrounded by his family, I couldn't help but reflect on how much I wished he had listened—how much I wished he could have seen the bigger picture and grasped the things we tried to share with him.

Ultimately, it became evident that he wasn't really paying attention. He ignored the warnings, the love, the guidance. It's a difficult reality, one that I wish wasn't so evident. It served as a reminder of how crucial it is to truly listen—not only to those around us but to the essence of life itself. We may not always have the opportunity to try again, and our inability to truly listen can lead to significant consequences.

Standing before Zack's casket, I was overwhelmed by a profound sense of loss, yet there was also a weight of responsibility that settled in my heart. I gently placed a cross on his chest and softly whispered, "Now, you are with God in peace." That moment held deep meaning. Zack faced many challenges throughout his life, but in that moment, I could see he had found his rest—his peace. The cross represented not only faith but also a deep sense of hope. It served as a reminder that, no matter what he had faced, he was now embraced by a higher power, liberated from the burdens he had endured for so long. Although I felt the heaviness of his loss, there was also a feeling of resolution, understanding that he had finally discovered the tranquility that had been absent during his life.

That moment with Zack, that cross on his chest, opened my eyes to the importance of truly listening. At times, the challenges we face in life can convey profound messages. Zack's journey was marked by his struggle; his difficulty in listening and genuinely understanding others took him to a place from which he couldn't find his way back. It caused me to think about the significance of truly listening—to take a moment, to pause, and to understand not only the words but the feelings that lie beneath them.

I reflected on how much suffering might have been spared if he had truly listened and embraced the lessons that life was presenting to him. But I also came to understand that this lesson wasn't solely for him—it was meant for all of us.

I've always felt that our challenges hold valuable lessons for us, as long as we're open to hearing them. Zack's story, while deeply moving, serves as a poignant reminder of the importance of heeding the insights offered by others, by life experiences, and by our own inner voice. Life often doesn't offer us second chances, and when we get swept up in the need to justify ourselves, defend our choices, or prove our point, we overlook the valuable lessons that could foster our growth. Real growth occurs when we truly listen—not only to those around us but also to the quiet insights that arise from within, from the calmness of our own hearts.

Zack's passing serves as a heartfelt reminder of the significance of seeking understanding. When we cease to listen, we cease to grow. When we cease to learn, we cease to grow. It's important to go beyond simply hearing words; we need to truly listen with the aim of understanding and embracing the lessons that life presents to us. At times, the lessons we learn are wrapped in experiences of pain, loss, or struggle. When we open ourselves to truly hearing others, we can transform those experiences into opportunities for growth, becoming more understanding and caring individuals.

Zack's death will forever leave a profound impact on my heart. In his memory, I decide to pay closer attention—to life, to those around me, and to my own feelings. I prefer to take the time to understand before I react or explain myself. From my experience of losing Zack, I've come to realize that genuine listening is essential for growth, healing, and grasping the profound lessons life presents. Life has a unique way of communicating with us, especially during tough times, but it requires us to be open and receptive.

As I reach the conclusion of this journey, I find myself reflecting on all that has influenced me—the peaks and valleys, the victories and the challenges. Each lesson I've shared and every story I've told reflects my true self and the person I aspire to be. By sharing my truth with you, I aim to help others grasp the profound pain and growth that life entails; I'm also reflecting on the journey I've taken to arrive at this point. It may have its challenges and imperfections, but it truly belongs to me.

The experiences I've gone through—pain, love, loss, and redemption—have truly influenced my beliefs and my sense of purpose. I've come to realize that life isn't measured by what we collect, but by the connections we create and the love we share. We all belong to a greater whole beyond our individual selves. The things we do, the decisions we make, and the things we say create waves in the world, impacting those around us, even if we're not aware of it. Ultimately, what truly matters is the love we give, the principles we stand by, and the impact we create for those who come after us.

Yet, there's an additional desire I hold. It goes beyond my own tranquility, or even the tranquility of those dear to me. I truly hope for a world filled with peace. I envision a time when love transcends mere conversation and becomes a powerful force that we all wholeheartedly embrace. A moment when individuals truly hear one another, strive to comprehend, and respond with kindness instead of apprehension. A moment when we embrace the positive in one another, regardless of our imperfections and variations. I understand this might seem like a far-fetched idea, but I truly think it's attainable. I truly think that everyone has a part to contribute in bringing it to life.

As we wrap up this chapter, I want to share something important: true peace begins from within. To transform the world, we need to begin with our own personal growth. We should embrace self-love, practice active listening, offer forgiveness, and approach others with kindness. It's through this connection that we can extend our love to others, fostering peace within our communities, our nations, and eventually, the entire world. It begins with each of us, and as we choose to embody love and peace, that energy will naturally radiate outward. A single individual has the power to transform the world, beginning with a single choice, a simple action, or a heartfelt moment of love.

I truly believe that one day, we can create a world where peace is not just something we wish for, but something we actually experience. I look forward to a time when we can put aside our differences and focus on uplifting one another. I wish for us to truly listen, to grasp things more completely, and to love wholeheartedly. The journey to that world might be lengthy, yet each step is truly valuable. If this book inspires even a single person to take that initial step, then it will have been truly worthwhile.

As I complete this journey and think about everything I've experienced, I want to share something meaningful with you—something I hope you take along as you move forward on your own path. I hope for you, and for everyone, this:

"Real peace starts within an individual and radiates out to touch the lives of others. Love is the seed, and peace is what we harvest"

Let's sow the seeds of love today, as they will blossom into the harvest of peace tomorrow.
    Tanner Bergsma
    Global Advocate for Peace and Love

Tanner Bergsma is an inspiring autistic author, entrepreneur, and activist dedicated to helping others find the light in the darkness. Through their work, Tanner transforms personal experiences of overcoming adversity into a mission to empower individuals and create meaningful change.

A compassionate storyteller and advocate, Tanner's writing blends motivation and practical guidance, offering readers the tools to navigate challenges and discover their inner strength. With a focus on inclusivity, housing, mental health, and accessibility, Tanner develops innovative solutions to systemic barriers, ensuring support for those who need it most. Driven by a passion for resilience and human connection, Tanner's work lights the way for others to rise above their struggles and embrace their brightest potential.

www.ingramcontent.com/pod-product-compliance
Lightning Source LLC
Jackson TN
JSHW071537190125
77308JS00001B/1